The Life Inside:
A Christian Woman's Perspective

Copyright © 2010 by Tara Jackson

All Rights Reserved

ISBN 1453628339

Contents

This book is lovingly dedicated to my husband, Luke. Thank you, Luke for loving me, caring for me and believing in me. This book and my life would not be what it is without your love, prayer and support.
I love you.

Introduction

As you begin the journey of pregnancy there is so much to learn about yourself and the world around you. You will learn things about your body that you have never known before. You will learn how you handle being pregnant, as well as how to take care of the life inside you. It is truly amazing that God has created our bodies to carry a child safely and yet so delicately. I still stand in amazement each day as I look back at both of my pregnancies.

When you find out you are pregnant, if you were planning for a child or if you were hoping for one, you are usually ecstatic at the news. Some of you may not have been expecting to be pregnant, but are ready now to embrace the new challenge. So now that you have gotten over the *"Oh my goodness, I'm pregnant"* and reality has set in let's move into the reason for this book.

You start to realize that you are completely responsible for this child. You begin to think about what should I eat, what should I drink, and how do I feel. You begin to realize that you are more tired and that you are hungry at different times during the day than before. You realize that you are not able to eat as much at normal meal times or that you have to eat little snacks in between meals. You realize that the life you once knew has drastically changed. For some people this brings great joy and excitement, but for others it brings fear and anxiety. Most women will face some fear and anxiety, but some will face some very real struggles and thoughts that are just from Satan. The devil tries to steal the joy of having a life inside you. Women, we are the only ones who will know what it feels like to have a life inside us. We are the precious chosen ones to feel the kicking, the moving and the continuous hiccups. We continue to watch our bodies do phenomenal things and go back to "normal." Don't be surprised at body changes. Our bodies are made to do this. Our bodies are made to do it without intervention. I have had two children, one by induction with epidural assistance and one naturally, at midwifery center, in a birthing tub. I can say that both were the most amazing experiences. The fact that your body can do what it needs to in order to deliver a baby is nothing short of a miracle. I have never experienced a C-section and, quite frankly, after talking with family and friends who have experienced them, I am happy I never did. Those of you who have or will in the future, God is still the author of that life inside you. You are still going to have a child at the end of the day and that is the focus to remember.

Now, for the pregnancy: you will get hungry, constipated, happy, sad, scared, joyous, nervous and elated. There are so many emotions that will overtake you. You may be a crier by God's design, but you find yourself crying more. You may not be a crier, but you find yourself crying and thinking, "What is wrong with me?" You are made with emotions that will shock you! God has created each of us with the ability to have emotions. Let us embrace them in every situation of life. This amazing nine month period that you are in, want to be in or have been in, is a cherished and predestined time that God has for you. Each pregnancy is different, and each pregnancy is wonderful, even in the midst of challenges. Some women have experienced what they would say are hard pregnancies and some easy. Those hard ones have taught those women how to let go and let God have control. Some women plan out their exact delivery from the time of labor to the time of delivery. Let me be the first to burst that bubble. The baby will come when God says, "Now my child is your moment, go and meet your Mommy and Daddy and do what I have planned for you". That moment when the baby arrives is indescribable. We long for this moment during the entire pregnancy. We desire to see the face of a person we know exists, but has not yet entered this world. We want to hold our child, kiss our child and tell our child we love them. That time will come. While you are pregnant, love that child, talk to that child, but most of all pray for that child. Pray for the desires of that child's heart to be met, pray for God's hand of protection to be upon them all the days of their life (Psalm 91). Pray that God will guide you and your spouse everyday that you have with this child and that you may direct them in the ways of the Father. We must remember that we are merely His earthly authority over this child. HE IS THE ONE WHO HAS IT ALL FIGURED OUT, so trust Him. I encourage each of you while you are in the hospital or home, the first chance you get as a family after your delivery, to dedicate that child to the Lord by saying,

> *"Father, this child is yours from this moment on. We let go and let You have Your way with him/her. We pray that You will guide and direct us every step of the way. We pray that You will show us as the child is in our care what is best for him/her. We pray You will help us nurture the child to strive after Your will. Please have control and please have Your hand of protection and love upon him/her, Amen."*

It really makes a difference when you give your children to the Lord. The worry and fear goes away after you turn them over unto His hands and trust Him. Begin to listen today to His leading. Being a parent is a forever thing; no turning back now. Once you have been pregnant, you are a parent and will be forever. Being a parent had always scared me a bit, but God showed me that we are His children and He is fond of us all. He has control so I must let go of my children and trust that He has control. How hard yet how easy is this concept? The hard part is actually grasping it, but the doing it tends to be easier as we trust His best for them!

Take care of yourself while you are pregnant. Eat right, drink water and get rest. Your body is doing an amazing work. If you are extremely tired, then rest. If you are hungry, eat healthy. Your body is in such a different place than normal, so pay attention to it.

Chapter 1

I am pregnant, Now What?

Now that you are pregnant and that you have nine months of this new lifestyle, what do you do with all the decisions you have to make during this time? There are decisions like what room in the house will become the nursery, what colors do we want, do we want to find out the gender of the baby, what name should we choose, and the list of decisions continues. When you get to the point where you can find out the gender of the baby, assuming you will find out, don't worry what others think because this is your time to enjoy. You will make these decisions. Just remember, if people are asking you how you are all the time or if they can do anything for you, just know that they love you, they care and that is why they are always asking. You can feel smothered, but remember the people who are in your immediate family are getting a new addition as well. It is okay to make boundaries with them if needed. There are several books available about boundaries and they each share with you healthy ways to have relational boundaries with family and friends. Having and putting boundaries in place can be difficult; however, it is very necessary with some relationships. This time of your life is precious, so enjoy it!

The inevitable name selection process can be so dramatic. Many people get bent out of shape about this decision. If you choose to tell others then tell them. If you choose not to tell people, then don't, but do it kindly and respectfully. The people in your life need to respect your decision. They don't have to like it, but they need to respect it. I always wanted to know the gender of our children and I always had them named before we would find out the gender. We had both a boy's name and a girl's name. From the day we found out, we called the child by name. As for me, it provided a feeling of being closer to the child as if we were already connecting with them. People would ask, "What if you change your mind on the name?" I simply responded, "Then we changed the name." If it happened, then it happened. Not a big deal. We always looked up the meaning and made sure we liked what the name meant before we named them, but beyond that, we just named the child based on what we felt was a great name or a name we liked. We didn't make a huge deal out of it. It is amazing to see how people around you will put themselves in your life all of the sudden because something life changing is happening to you. This is really strange for some people. I never minded it because I knew that these people have been down the path I was traveling and they truly had my best interest at heart. I am not saying that you need to take every word they say as truth or as the final word, just listen and separate the advice. Separate good advice from bad, based on your belief system. I firmly believe that what I say has a direct effect on what takes place in my life. The Bible warns us about the use of our tongues and the words that are spoken. I read Scriptures more carefully and realized that we do have the ability to speak blessing or cursing upon our lives and our children. Which do you want to be a part of in your life? You have the power and control over what you say, choose to speak life.

Chapter 2

Bad Reports

In the case of a bad report from the doctor, or ultrasound, DON'T DWELL ON THE BAD REPORT! Whose report do you believe? My husband and I chose to believe God's Word over the doctors. We are thankful for the doctors and appreciate all they know and all that they do to provide information. The facts are to be viewed as a blessing because they show us exactly how and what to pray for or pray against. The information that the doctors provide is factual. The fact is what they say. Truth can always change fact. We believe God's Word as truth, so we took God's Word as our final truth, and therefore we watched in great expectation, our facts change and line up with His truth. We are created in His image. We believe in the True Physician and the One who gave the doctors their knowledge.

We went into the ultrasound certain our baby was perfect. We were certain we were having a boy. We went for our 20 week ultrasound and the tech said, "Do you want to know the sex of the baby?" "YES," we yelled! The words we have been waiting to hear for 20 plus weeks: "IT"S A GIRL!" she said. What! We were shocked! We just knew we were having a boy. We were certain. God gave us a girl. Our first daughter was perfect. She was growing exactly as fast as she was supposed to be based on her gestational age. We were living in Italy at the time, so we were without family nearby and we were so thankful for our friends that we had made during our time there. One couple especially impacted our lives. My best friend was pregnant with her second child and her baby was due four days before mine. What a blessing to be pregnant at the same time as your best friend! We shared everything with each other, from cravings to emotions. She was one who had received a bad report at an ultrasound. They said that their baby had fluid around her heart and they needed to do further testing. We opened up the Word of God, and immediately started praying and believing God was going to provide healing for that little baby. We prayed and we prayed for her. They went to deliver her and she was perfect! The Word of God has power.

When I was pregnant with our second child, we again were determined it was a boy and that the ultrasound would show the baby perfectly healthy and normal. So we go into the ultrasound, and the tech said, "Do you want to know the sex of the baby?" "YES," we exclaimed! She said, "IT"S A GIRL!" What! We were shocked! Unbelievable! We were again certain it was a boy! It was funny really. We then went through the rest of the ultrasound and the words you never want to hear, "Let me look at that again, I see something abnormal." The thought that came to my mind was, "Well, I hope so, there is a baby in there," as I giggled out of nervousness and fear. The ultrasound tech could see that there was what she called a "bright bowel". A bright bowel can be from early bleeding in pregnancy, a sign of Down's syndrome and probably an array of other reasons. The ultrasound tech and doctor wanted us to go receive a high risk ultrasound as a follow-up. What a damper on such a precious moment. We loved our baby girl regardless of the bad report and would accept her how she was given, but we knew the power of the Word of God and what it says. We made the appointment and went to the high risk ultrasound. My friend from church was the ultrasound technician. God is good to have blessed us with our friend doing this ultrasound. We were already quite nervous, so knowing that the technician was our friend provided additional comfort to us. She too saw the bright bowel and then said the words you never want to hear, "I see something else that is questionable." My exact thoughts were, "Are you serious?" followed with a sarcastic tone. We went into that appointment knowing the tech was going to say the bright bowel was gone! We did not expect her to tell us that not only was the bright bowel still there, but also a large nuchal fold. The nuchal fold is where the back of the neck was measuring larger and more thick than normal. That too, is a sign for Down's syndrome. At that point, I fell completely apart. I freaked out momentarily while lying there at the ultrasound. The doctor offered to provide us the advice of a genetics counselor. My husband wanted to see the genetics counselor, because he is a statistics, numbers kind of guy. I, however, am not a numbers kind of girl and no numbers would be fine with me! So I just tried to keep my thoughts focused on something else while the genetics counselor provided all the statistics and information. After meeting with the genetics counselor my husband was encouraged when we left, and I was heartbroken. I was not ok with this situation. I was scared out of my mind. I started saying in my mind, "How on earth was I supposed to do this? Why was this happening to us? I can't handle this Lord. What is going on?" I immediately called my mom because she was praying for the ultrasound to be clear of problems as well. She said, "It is okay, we know God's Word, but you need to dig into it more. Find scriptures that comfort you and build your faith." Wow, thanks Mom. Those words have forever changed my life. Needless to say, I had a lot of research to do because when it came to this situation I had no idea how to pray. As we tried to eat dinner that night, I just felt helpless and responsible. What did I do to make this happen? Did I do too much during the first half of pregnancy? So, that night I prayed and prayed and prayed. The next few days I spent searching the Word of God. I found many scriptures that helped me. I wrote them out and read them daily. I prayed for her healing and I came to the point in my faith to be able to say, "She is healed." I continued, "God, if I could only touch you, she would be healed." The account in the Bible of the women with the issue of blood came to mind (Luke 8:43-47). This time my faith was for my unborn child, one who does not know what faith is yet, one who hasn't even taken her first breath.

So I prayed:

"God, please heal her, have mercy and grace. Forgive me of my sins that make it possible for there to be imperfection. Oh my Savior, Jehovah Rophe, The Lord my Healer, I ask in faith, heal my daughter. I know your Word says that by Your stripes she is healed. I know that You bore our shame and sin that we may have life and have it abundantly! Oh God, I come in simple and little faith, as heartbroken and sad as I am, please help me keep the faith that knows and believes that YOU HAVE HEALED HER!"

Your faith has to go from believing that God CAN heal to knowing that He has ALREADY healed us when He died on the cross. The faith to believe that she was healed came after hours and days of praying, weeping, reasoning with God, and reading God's Word. I talked with Him about how to grow my faith through Scripture and how to stand when you feel like you have done everything to stand (Ephesians 6:10-20). I found many scriptures that gave me peace and you will find many of these in Chapter 7.

Chapter 3

Is this really my body?
I don't feel like myself.

How a woman feels about herself while pregnant will greatly determine the joy and happiness that she experiences. During pregnancy, your body will change so much and you may begin to wonder if this will ever end. You will go from knowing your body to being completely thrown into a body that is trying to figure itself out. You can experience nausea and in a short period of time gain an abundance of energy. You can be happy and the next minutes become sad. Your emotions will appear to go from here to there and your feelings are sensitive and tender. I remember thinking when pregnant with my first daughter that I could not wait to wear maternity clothes and hope I do not gain too much weight. If you think about why you will need to wear maternity clothes you may laugh as it is directly related to the fact that you are gaining weight.

HELP! I'm gaining weight!

Gaining weight in pregnancy is important and normal, but does not give you a free ticket to gain too much weight. Some women gain a majority of their weight in the beginning and taper off in the second trimester. At the end of the pregnancy in most cases it will simply just equal out. The important thing to remember is eating healthy while giving yourself some grace to have a snack of choice periodically and to stay reasonably active. The truth is that you will gain weight in pregnancy. We must come to grips with that reality. Our society, as well as our own added pressure, has made gaining even one pound a negative thing. I am not condoning obesity, but am saying that too many women are hard on themselves and start to live in fear that they are going to be overweight because of pregnancy.

During my first pregnancy, I started out with normal weight gain. I was already heavier than what was normal according to the doctor's charts and scales, but by the end of the pregnancy had only gained 25 pounds total. You might be thinking that is a lot or you might think that is great for weight gain during pregnancy. My doctor was thrilled with a total of 25 pounds. You must consider the way your body changes. The top of your body gets larger, your middle gets bigger and your body will rapidly change like no other time in your life. The truth is that you are going to gain weight. Do not stress about this! Our culture has put too much pressure on women and their bodies during and after pregnancy. Your body is created to carry this child.

We must love ourselves and love how our bodies are designed in order to stay in a place of true happiness and joy. Weight gain comes and goes during and after pregnancy. I am not saying let yourself go and not take care of yourself, but love who you are and work with what you have been given. Thank God for creating your body this way. You are an amazing creation!

The Rollercoaster Ride!!!

After the delivery of my first daughter, I went through an emotional rollercoaster and through many issues, as every new mother does. I did not tell anyone about the feelings I was experiencing. I did not tell my husband about these problems nor did I allow him to help me. I kept it all inside.

We lived in Italy at the time, so with no family around, things seemed to get darker each day. I focused feelings more inwardly and not on anyone or anything else. I loved my husband and my new daughter. I loved what God was doing and where He had placed us at this particular time in our lives. I praise God for our friends during this time. We grew very close to many of our friends, but there was one couple that helped more than they will ever know. The daily grind involved being home with my new child, but something wasn't right deep on the inside. I was unhappy within myself and felt like I just was not good enough, not a good mother, nor a good wife and had weight that was not there before pregnancy.

My weight began to increase beyond what it was before pregnancy. Exercising was not helping. I was beginning to feel that I did not love myself for who I was created to be and the weight would not go down. My life was totally out of balance. I loved my husband and daughter with everything I had within me, but I could not stand myself or the person that had I become after pregnancy. The worst thing about not loving yourself is that you cannot get away from yourself. You live in yourself constantly. I felt sad and if I was being completely honest with myself, I knew that I was depressed. I knew it. I did not want to admit it and digging even deeper I realized I was afraid of it. I did not want to be humiliated or embarrassed because of it.

I experienced suicidal tendencies and thoughts. I had feelings of regret, fear and anger. I did not understand how my best friend could look into her newborn baby's eyes and be in love. It saddened me that I was not feeling that way. I WANT TO CLARIFY – THIS HAD NOTHING TO DO WITH MY DAUGHTER! She was and is perfect; she is special and a true blessing in my life. This was my issue and did not stem from her at all! This kind of depression is something that affects some women after pregnancy. Know that it is not your child that you are sad or depressed about if you struggle with postpartum depression. Mayo Clinic defines postpartum depression as a more severe form of emotional distress. You have to get out of that pit. You cannot stay there and be healthy. I lived in the darkest part of that pit for a full year. It took another year and a half to love myself enough to function in a semi normal way. I started to love myself for who I was and not what I looked like or didn't look like. I not only had to go to the Word of God, but I had to trust and believe the Word of God! Honestly it was during my second pregnancy that I truly began to love myself and care about myself without reservation.

During my second pregnancy I was having fainting spells. It was horrible and scary. All of the sudden I would go into tunnel vision and then pass out. Other times I was back to normal a few minutes later. After several episodes I finally consulted with my doctors. I went and had heart tests and blood work done. They figured out it was my iron level. I was border line anemic. My body was greatly impacted by my low iron level. My doctor started me on iron supplement pills and my levels began to rise to normal levels. I realized that I also had choices to make. I needed to stop taking in as much sugar. Each of these helped stabilize the episodes and I began feeling 'normal' again. My second pregnancy was wonderful and scary all in the same. You may be questioning how it was wonderful and scary. The answer: I loved the fact that I was carrying a child; I loved feeling life inside of me and her hiccups at exactly 8pm every

night. The scary part was the passing out, the feeling
of weakness because of that, and the bad reports of
Down's syndrome. I began searching the scriptures
regarding my daughter's healing and the Lord led me
back to Psalm 139. I was reading and meditating on
this scripture for our daughter's spiritual, mental,
physical and emotional health. The Lord showed me
that it was for my health also. He wanted me to know
that when and if I would love myself because He loved
me so much, that things would change. I would lose
the weight that I had gained, I would feel better about
myself, and I would desire to exercise and eat in a
healthier manner. I can tell you this worked, because
of the balance that I gave to my life.

I came to the end of my pregnancy and had my
appointment with the mid-wife, and the looming scale
was staring me in the face. I got on the scale, and the
verdict: 5 pounds of total weight gain. OH MY WORD!
WHAT! I had actually lost weight during pregnancy!
Just like going into my first pregnancy, I had some

weight to lose. I was too heavy at the beginning and by the end when I delivered my little girl, I left the hospital 25 pounds less than when I started the pregnancy. I am like any other female and yes, that was a highlight for me. I knew that it was up to me from that point on to stay healthy. I felt like God gave me a great jump start and it was up to me to continue what He began.

The Change to Healthy Living!!!!

As I began the journey of living a healthier lifestyle, the desires I had always had of running and completing a race were at the forefront of my thoughts. I know that sounds kind of childish, but I have always wanted to run a race. So my husband and I began to "train" for a race. We signed up for a 5K and created a training schedule. We would take turns running in the evenings and we would eat a little differently. The day of the race came. I was nervous and concerned that I would not be able to do it. With the love of my husband and two of his co-workers, we ran it and finished it. I ran it in 42 minutes and that was an awesome feeling. I crossed that finish line and started crying uncontrollably as I threw my arms around my daughter. I couldn't believe I did it. I met a life long goal and I was four months post delivery! It felt wonderful. I felt great. I felt like I could accomplish anything. I realized, at that point, that God had given me the Word to read and meditate on so that I would love myself enough to try to accomplish any goal I had; that in turn helped me understand that taking a little time out for me was so rewarding.

Let us revisit the weight thing for a moment: love yourself where you are and if you feel you weigh more than you should or would like to, LOVE YOURSELF TO THE WEIGHT YOU SHOULD BE AT! Do not go down the path of kicking yourself, being mad at yourself or thinking you have done something wrong. Just start by loving yourself. Give yourself a break and give yourself some love. If you are pregnant and feel that you are gaining weight too fast or that you are heavier than what you thought while pregnant, ask your doctor and do something to change your circumstance. If your doctor says you that you should do something to not gain so fast, do what they say. If your doctor says it is normal, then let it be. Do what you know is right: eat healthy, exercise (according to what you should do during pregnancy, do NOT over do it) and stay in the Word of God. That is how you are going to be able to love yourself through the changes that your body will inevitably make. Those things will happen, embrace them and love them. There is help where you need it. Ask for help if you need help. Do not hesitate because of fear, embarrassment or humiliation. It is far greater to get out of the mind slump than stay in it. It takes a lot of effort to get out once you are there. Trust in the Lord with all your heart! He created you, He knows you and He loves you. Let Him be your guide, comfort and companion. Be honest with Him and yourself!

Chapter 4

Is it okay that I worry?

Not at all! Just because you are in a situation, in this case pregnancy, you are not given a free ticket to start worrying. Worrying is ineffective!

During your pregnancy, you can start to worry about unnecessary things. People are anxious to give you their opinion and their experiences, some positive and some negative. Now, I am not faulting anyone for doing this. I happen to be one of these people myself. You just get so excited for the person and want to share with them. My sister-in-law was pregnant with her first baby and I told her so much information that she was probably completely overwhelmed after talking to me! You just desire for people to not go through the things you went through or if it was a good experience, you want that for them as well. It is amazing what God can teach you while pregnant. When you finally have the baby in your arms, you realize that your life changes forever. It is a great thing! It is important to be prepared for those changes.

If you are pregnant with your first child there will be a lot of learning involved. Once you have a child, you begin learning for the rest of your life. The initial "OH MY WORD! I NOW HAVE A BABY--- WHERE IS THE MANUAL?" that will hit, can be counteracted with peace and calmness. You need to remember to stay focused on this little life and try to let God lead you. It is extremely important to keep your time with the Lord. Daily time with HIM is critical. He helps you throughout your day. He gives you peace when you lay your head down at night, and then when you are up again in a few hours. He gives you the strength that you NEED as the parent of a newborn or the pregnant woman who has to go to the bathroom every hour of the night. The nights that you see the clock at 1, 2, 3, 4, 5, 6 and then get up at 7! He helps sustain you. He gives you the strength and ability to persevere. It is only by Him! Worry is not of God, so do not give yourself the opportunity to fall into the trap of worry. Surround yourself with family and friends that keep you positive and focused on Christ. Do things that keep you positive like taking a walk, or taking a nap. The most important thing you can do is to keep your mind on His Word.

Chapter 5

My Quiet time turned into Glider time

I really fell into this trap of "my time" and how was "I" suppose to have time with the Lord; the traditional "quiet time" that I needed? I called my Mom, and asked her how on earth you are supposed to sit down quietly for an allotted amount of time with a newborn and all the other responsibilities in your home or at your job? She reminded me that praising Him is an act of worship. Praying is an act of worship and that rearing this child/these children are acts of worship. Yes, it is important to have "in the Word" time, *but* remember that in the Word time comes in many forms. Write them on index cards and put them around your house, your baby's nursery, your bathroom, stick them to the arm of your glider, etc. Places you know you will be so that when you are in those rooms/places you can read them and memorize them and dwell on them. This is writing them on the tablets of your heart (Prov. 3:3 NIV) like the Bible tells us to do. When we dwell and meditate on the Scripture, it is written on the tablets of our hearts. If there is a day where you physically can't open the Bible, have it in your heart so that you can meditate on it! You can pray while feeding the baby, changing a diaper and even disciplining a child; you master those things as time goes on. You can praise Him through song and through words of praise while doing other things.

It is wonderful to sing to Him and your child usually likes it as well. Getting the Word inside of you is important and do not let condemnations (Romans 8:1 NIV) take a hold of you because you are finding it hard to open the Word. Get the Word on Tape/CD/DVD or iPod and listen to it. Have it playing in your home. This will keep the peace in your home as well.

Focusing on the Lord is one thing that kept me from spiraling even further into depression. I can tell you that there were dark, dark, dark days; but the Word of God helped me see the truth and follow it out of that miserable, dark place. There are good days and there are bad days. The challenges that come during your day, battle them with the Word of God. You have to know the Word to use the Word! God will give you the wisdom, knowledge, understanding and discernment that you need in your everyday life. Pregnant or not, parent or not. He is always willing to give you what you need.

The Bible says, "You have not because you ask not." We need to ask him for wisdom. In James 1:5 the Word says, "He gives wisdom to all liberally and without reproach." He is willing, but we must ask. In Matthew 7:7 we are told, "Ask and you shall receive, seek and you shall find, knock and the door shall be opened unto you". He is ready and waiting, we just have to ask and receive. It is really that simple, but it is much harder as you are living it day in and day out. Ask someone to help you with this task; sit down and write down the verses that encourage you. Put them around your house and let God write them on your hearts. It makes all the difference. The importance of the Word of God in anyone's life is the foundation to a successful life. HIS WORD STANDS FIRM AND IS TRUTH! You can TRUST His word! It will not fail you!

Chapter 6

Is Postpartum Depression Real?

Now for the issue at hand: Is Postpartum Depression real? I have heard some pastors say that Christian women should not suffer from postpartum depression because they know Christ. Well, I am a Christian and I did suffer from postpartum depression. It happens to people and it happened to me. Now, I can give you the quick way of not falling into the trap and that is standing on the Word of God. The midwife I was seeing at the time of my second pregnancy told me that the probability of having postpartum again was more likely than it was the first time. The more pregnancies you have, the greater the risk for postpartum depression. I had scriptures laid out that I read every day while pregnant with my second child so that I would not fall into the trap of depression again. I was determined not to go through that a second time.

Mayo Clinic defines postpartum depression as a more severe form of emotional distress. I can say from experience that it is a very dark place. I will be honest and tell you that if you struggled or are struggling with this horrible problem, let me encourage you that YOU CAN/WILL RISE ABOVE with the help and love of the Holy Spirit. You can do this.

I would always think to myself that I wasn't good enough in all areas of my life, as a wife, mother, sister, daughter, aunt and friend. I was very self defeated and self abusive. My thoughts about myself were horrific. Death was an option that I thought about. Now tell me what on this earth is worth dying for? There are obviously things or people worth dying for but DEPRESSION is not one of them! This feeling can grip you and debilitate you and keep you so far from the arms of Christ. That is Satan's goal. His goal is to keep you from walking with Him and allowing Him to rescue you from this depression. Let Jesus rescue you. He already died for the depression and for your sorrows, so live in the restoration of joy and life. The chemicals in your body and the hormones in your body are given a big ride when you are pregnant and after pregnancy. Your body adjusts to these over a nine month period of time. Then all of the sudden the baby is delivered, everyone loves the baby and you are laying there tired, hungry, and feeling alone because the life that was inside of you is now in your arms. Remember you have been with another human, nonstop for nine months. It can feel very lonely. I know it can be hard. You can come out of this, but first, be honest with yourself, do not be condemned for admitting you are depressed. In Romans 8, we are told that, "There is now therefore no condemnation for those in Christ Jesus." Admit it and move on from it. Remember in the Bad Reports chapter when we discussed facts versus the truth? The fact is that you are depressed but the truth of God's Word is that you have the mind of Christ (1 Cor. 2:16). You do not have a spirit of fear, but of power, love and a sound mind (2

Tim. 1:7). You are healed. I know that none of us want to feel like we are admitting a "bad" thing, but if you do not admit it, you can not confront it. Do not wait until you are a year down the road like I was. Recognize the signs and deal with them. Some of the signs are clear and some are very indistinguishable with everyday emotions. In my case, the emotion of "feeling alone" was a major symptom. I wanted to be alone; I didn't mind if it is dark in the house; I wanted to stay in bed, or be in my pajamas all day. I didn't care if the things in the house pile up and up and up. I felt like life could go on without me and no one would miss me. THESE ARE LIES! DO NOT listen to them. They are not worth your time. God has you here at this time, for a purpose and a reason, and it is critical that you believe that. You can dwell in this depression, or dwell in His Word. You have to do the choosing. I am going to be pretty bold here and say something you probably won't like, and that is GET UP! The man by the pool of Bethesda was sick for over 30 years and all he had to do was GET UP! (John 5:1-9). God has given us the tools in His Word and by the Holy Spirit to get up and move on. We do not have to be a partaker in the realm of depression. Apply your faith and GET UP!

I remember telling my husband, that in Genesis it says that there will be pain in childbearing (Gen. 3:16), so what happened? There was pain in child bearing. May I take a minute to remind you that the pain in child bearing came along with the curse after the fall of mankind? We have the opportunity to live under the blessing of Jesus Christ, who wipes away the curse for us (Gal. 3:13 NIV and Duet. 28:1-14). Then with my second pregnancy, I realized that I was no longer under the curse of the pain of childbearing. I was under the blessing and Jesus had taken all the pain in childbearing and all the sorrow of postpartum when He died. I no longer had to dwell under that curse. I rebuked the curse and no longer walked in it. I finally got sick and tired of being sick and tired. The guy at the pool (Matt. 9:1-8 Amplified) finally had to make the choice to let go of the comfort of his disease. Yes, I said comfort. We can get so comfortable with where we are that we actually find ungodly peace and stay there. Why do you want to stay in a place where Satan keeps lying to you and telling you that you are not good, healthy or worth it? Rise up and walk. You have to walk in the power of the Holy Spirit. You have to be willing and desire to be well. You have to hear the Word, believe the Word in your heart, and by faith act on the Word (James 2:26 Amplified). I do not mean to just say, "Of course I want to be well." Put some action behind it. If you need to go to a doctor and get help, go. Do what is safe and what you need to do that will help you get out of it. Be honest with your significant other. It is critical that you tell him. If he doesn't understand, which you need to realize he probably won't because he isn't going through the same emotions as you, then tell him what you need. Tell him you need an extra hug that day, or need him to listen to your emotions and listen to you. He needs to be aware of what you are feeling so that you can have someone around you to hold you accountable. Be honest with yourself and with him. He loves you and he wants you to be healthy, believe me. He wants that woman that he fell in love with, not someone who doesn't care about herself and doesn't desire to take care of herself. He wants that same woman that desired to be a mother, to be a mother; not a person who just takes care of a baby; someone to engage with the children and someone to love and encourage as a mother. You are a mother whether you are pregnant or already have the baby. Remember that it is okay to feel these things and to feel overwhelmed, these are normal, just don't dwell there. Remember not to jump on the depression ship just because you are tired. You will be tired. You just gave birth. Your baby is hungry and the only way for your baby to communicate with you is through crying. He/she is just trying to tell you something. They do not know how to talk, so they cry. Try your best to not get frustrated because you are tired you can easily become upset. Give yourself some grace! You can feel scared and afraid. I don't mean, like "why didn't a manual come out with the baby" afraid, but just afraid. Even to this day I have a hard time explaining why I was afraid, or even what I was afraid of, but I was just afraid. "God has not given you a spirit of fear, but of power, love and a sound mind (2 Tim. 1:7 NIV)". "His grace is sufficient for you (2 Cor. 12:9)". Even if you can not explain yourself, confide in someone. Remember to at least admit your feelings so you can overcome them. We all have times when we are afraid or sad, as if someone frightened us or something horrible happens. These are not the times I am speaking of. The fear and sadness that can debilitate you and cause you to dwell in a pit that is dark and not healthy are the ones that I am addressing. This is a scary and lonely place. God desires us to rejoice in this time of life. If you find yourself swimming in these thoughts, talk to your husband, your doctor, or a friend. Let someone inside and know so they can help you. God will restore life to you. He will turn your sorrow into joy! It is said in 1 John 4:18 that, "There is no fear in love. But perfect love drives out fear, because fear has to do with punishment. The one who fears is not made perfect in love." Remember that God is love and we should rely on Him and in Him alone (1 John 4:16 NIV).

Chapter 7

Daily Scriptures for Daily Health

As I studied God's Word, I wrote these scriptures on index cards. The scriptures I spoke out loud and believed in my heart every day are:

Philippians 4: 6-7 NKJV
"Be anxious for nothing, but in everything by prayer and supplication, with thanksgiving, let your requests be made known to God; and the peace of God which surpasses all understanding will guard your hearts and minds through Christ Jesus!" NKJV

Philippians 4: 8-9 NKJV
"Finally brethren, whatever things are true, whatever things are noble, whatever things are just, whatever things are pure, whatever things are lovely, whatever things are of good report, if there is any virtue and if there is anything praise worthy-meditate on these things. The things which you learned and received and heard and saw in me, these do and the God of peace will be with you!"

Micah 7:7 NKJV
"Therefore I will look to the Lord; I will wait for the God on my salvation; My God will hear me!"

Philippians 1:6 NKJV
"...being confident of this very thing, that He who has begun a good work IN YOU will complete it until the day of Christ Jesus."

Psalm 139: 13-17 NKJV
"For you formed my inward parts; You covered me in my mother's womb. I will praise you for I am fearfully and wonderfully made, Marvelous are Your works, and that my soul knows very well. My frame was not hidden from you, when I was made in secret, and skillfully wrought in the lowest parts of the earth. Your eyes saw my substance, being yet unformed. And in your book they all were written, the days fashioned for me, when as yet there were none of them. How precious also are YOUR thoughts TO ME, O God! How great is the sum of them!"

Proverbs 29:25 NKJV
"The fear of man brings a snare, but whoever trusts in the Lord shall be safe!"

Hebrews 10:19-23 NKJV
"Therefore brethren having boldness to enter the Holiest by the blood of Jesus, by a new and living way which He consecrated for us through the veil that is His flesh, and having a High Priest over the house of

God, let us draw near with a true heart in FULL ASSURANCE of faith, having our hearts sprinkled from an evil conscience and our bodies washed with pure water. Let us holdfast the confession of our hope without wavering for He who Promised is faithful!"

Romans 8:39 NKJV
"Yet in all these things we are more than conquerors through Him who loved us."

Romans 8:28 NKJV
"And we know that all things work together for good to those who love God, to those who are the called according to His purpose."

Isaiah 53:4-5 NKJV
"Surely He has borne our griefs, and carried our sorrows, yet we esteemed Him stricken, smitten by God, and afflicted; BUT He was wounded for our transgressions, He was bruised for our iniquities; the chastisement for our peace was upon Him and by His stripes we are healed."

Proverbs 3:5-6 NKJV
"Trust in the Lord with all your heart, and lean not on your own understanding; but in all your ways acknowledge Him and He shall direct your paths."

Hebrews 2:4 NKJV
"God also bearing witness both with signs and wonders, with various miracles and gifts of the Holy Spirit according to HIS OWN WILL."

John 16:21-24 NKJV
"A woman, when she is in labor, has sorrow because her hour has come; but as soon as she has given birth to the child, she no longer remembers the anguish, for joy that a human being has been born into the world. Therefore you now have sorrow, but I will see you again and your hearts will rejoice, and your joy no one will take from you. And in that day you will ask Me nothing. Most assuredly, I say to you, whatever you ask the Father in My name, He will give you. Until now you have asked nothing in My Name, Ask, and you will receive that your joy may be full."

John 17:23 NKJV
"I in them, and you in Me; that they may be made perfect in one and that the world may know that You have sent Me, and have loved them as You have loved Me."

James 1:2 NKJV
"My brethren, count it all joy when you fall into various trials, knowing that the testing of your faith produces patience. But let patience have its perfect work, that you may be perfect and complete, lacking nothing."

Luke 1:42 NKJV

"Then she spoke with a loud voice and said, Blessed are you among women, and blessed is the fruit of your womb!"

Luke 1:45 NKJV

"Blessed is she who believed, for there will be a fulfillment of those things which were told her from the Lord."

Colossians 3:15 NKJV

"And let the peace of God rule in your hearts, to which also you were called in one body; and be thankful. Let the Word of Christ dwell in you richly in all wisdom teaching and admonishing one another in psalms and hymns and spiritual songs singing with grace in your hearts to the Lord."

Colossians 3:17 NKJV

"And whatever you do in word or deed do all in the name of the Lord Jesus, giving thanks to God the Father through Him."

2 Corinthians 13:9 NKJV

"For we are glad when we are weak and you are strong. And this also we pray, that you may be made complete."

2 Corinthians 13:11 NKJV
"Finally brethren, farewell, become complete. Be of good comfort, be of one mind, live in peace, and the God of love and peace will be with you."

James 1:17-18 NIV
"Every good and perfect gift is from above, coming down from the Father of the heavenly lights, who does not change like shifting shadows, He chose to give us birth through the word of truth that we might be the kind of first fruits of all he created."

Chapter 8

Belief

I believed whole-heartedly that my daughter was going to be perfect and complete, lacking nothing! Ten weeks later we had another ultrasound, and my friend was the technician again. She believed with us that we would see a perfectly healthy little one. My husband and I agreed on the first name, but we were still debating over the middle name.

I wanted Joy to be her middle name as I believed that the "joy of the Lord was my strength". That is the only way I was making it through the days until we had another ultrasound. The tech came in and performed the ultrasound. "Well", she says, "The bright bowel is gone. Let's check everything else." She measured her bones, thickness of her arms and legs, her nasal bone, etc. After awhile I said, "Have we checked the neck?" She said, "I am going there now." As we waited in anticipation for what she would say, she looked over and had a tear in her eye. She said, "Tara, she is perfect. The nuchal fold is measuring normal. She is right where she needs to be!" OH MY WORD, A CRY FEST WAS GOING ON!! My God is faithful! He is awesome! Praise God from whom all blessings flow! My daughter is perfect. My friend gave us a few minutes with her on the screen while she left the room. We looked at her on the computer screen and cried. My husband said, "The JOY of the Lord is our strength. God is good!" He said, "Her middle name needs to be Joy!" Praise His name forever!

After we had a moment of pure gratitude and gave thanks to our Father for His goodness, we finished the appointment and headed to go pick up our oldest from her grandmother's house. We called our moms (who most of the time, are our messengers) and told them the fantastic news about their granddaughter. It was so wonderful. It is truly amazing to feel and sense what God can do. When you actually have a situation in your life and He takes care of it, you realize what a mighty God we serve!

We need to remember that faith is huge in this whole process of conceiving, pregnancy and post-delivery. It takes faith to know that He is calling you into such a wonderful position as becoming a parent. It is as challenging and as it is rewarding. It can be at times tiring, but it is uplifting. It is constant and a huge responsibility. When we become parents He gives us the grace, the love and the capacity to handle being a parent. He doesn't just give a child to you and say, "Here you go, have fun and do it right!" His grace abounds daily. He loves us so much that He rewards us with children and He trusts us with them. We are responsible to take care of these children in this world. We are to make sure their earthly needs are met, but He guides us, directs us, protects us, and provides for us. We must seek Him daily to know His desires for us and our children. We have to always remember that

our children are HIS CHILDREN, and we are just responsible for them on earth. We should seek out what the Word says about rearing children and what it truly takes to do it in a Godly way. It takes faith, perseverance, character, love, and so much more. I have learned so much and understand so much about 1 Corinthians 13 just by being a parent. When our daughter's came into our lives God's grace was far more abundant.

When life happens we need to remember that God will stay with us. He isn't going to leave us and He isn't going to forsake us (Hebrews 13:5 NIV). He will stand by us as long as we allow Him in our lives. Believing that He can do all things is simplistic, but believing He will do it for you personally is faith.

Conclusion

I pray that you have learned that God is always with you. I pray that these scriptures will encourage you. I pray that you can write them down, put them around your home, in your car and anywhere else you think you need to put them. When you do this you surround yourself with His Word. I know that He is able to do anything you need Him to do; you just have to ask, believe and receive.

I pray you find that God is your strength. God is your help and He loves you. He created you in His image. Remember through all the changes your body faces during pregnancy and all the emotional changes you feel, that God created YOU. He made you with a mind, with a will and with emotions. Use them for His glory. He is faithful to help you in times of trouble and in times of need. You are beautiful, special and valuable. Motherhood is an amazing gift. He has freely given, freely receive it today.

Works Cited

www.mayoclinic.com/health/postpartum-depression/ds00546 June 7, 2008. 1998-2010 MFMER